All About
PREVENTING FALLS

By Laura Flynn R.N., B.N., M.B.A., in consultation with her nurse educator associates and physicians who assisted in contributing and editing.

ISBN No: 978 1 896616 62 9

The publisher, Mediscript Communications Inc., acknowledges the financial support of the Government of Canada through the Canadian Book Fund for our publishing activities.

Printed in Canada

www.mediscript.net

Book and Front Cover design by:
Brian Adamson, www.AdamsonGraphics.net

PF1002011

ALL ABOUT BOOKS
Trusted • Reliable • Certified

- 40+ titles available
- Comply with accreditation and regulatory bodies
- Suitable for caregivers, boomers with elderly parents, health workers, auxiliary health staff & patients
- Self study style with "test yourself" section
- Health On the Net (HON) certified

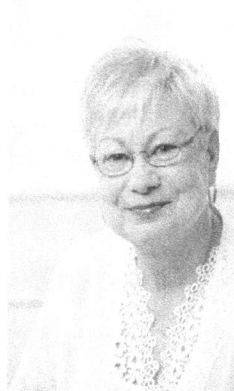

Some of our titles:

Alzheimers Disease	Arthritis	Multiple Sclerosis
Pain	Strokes	Elder Abuse
Falls Prevention	Incontinence	Nutrition & Aging
Personal Care	Positioning	Confusion
Transferring people	Care of the Back	Skin Care

For complete list of titles go to www.mediscript.net

Contact: 1 800 773 5088
Fax 1800 639 3186 • Email: mediscript30@yahoo.ca

CONTENTS

INTRODUCTION

This book provides basic, non controversial and trusted information that can help a wide spectrum of readers.

The primary objective of the information is to help a person provide effective quality care to a loved one or someone in his or her care.

Your role as a caregiver could mean the older person in your care is a family member or loved one, or you may be a non family member who is helping out a friend. Alternatively, you may be a paid health worker providing quality care for a client. With this in mind, we will alternate between referring to family members, loved ones, older persons and clients.

All the information is reliable and was written by a group of eminent nurse educators who ensured the information complies with best practice guidelines and satisfies the various accreditation and regulatory bodies. Because there is so much unreliable information on the internet, you can be assured the "All About" publications are HON (Health On the Net) certified.

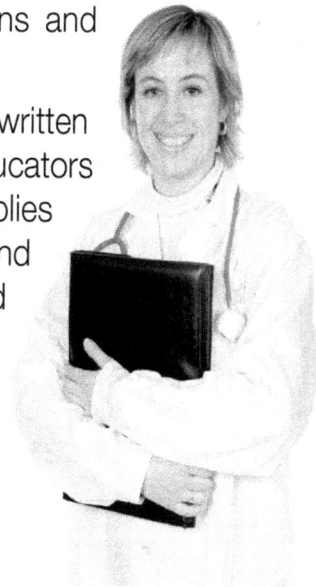

This book can be an invaluable aid to:

- A caregiver caring for a relative or friend;
- A health worker seeking a reference aid;
- An older patient or person at risk of falling;
- Any person involved in health care wishing to expand his or her knowledge.

SOMETHING TO THINK ABOUT...

One never notices what has been done; one can only see what remains to be done.

Marie Curie

AN IMPORTANT MESSAGE FROM THE PUBLISHER

Each person's treatment, advice, medical aids, physical therapy and other approaches to health care are unique and highly dependant upon the diagnosis and overall assessment by the medical team.

We emphasize therefore that the information within this book is not a substitute for the advice and treatment from a health care professional.

This book provides generic information concerning the issues around falls and common sense, well-established care practices for people who are at risk of falling.

With all this in mind, the publishers and authors disclaim any responsibility for any adverse effects resulting directly or indirectly from the suggestions contained within this book or from any misunderstanding of the content on the part of the reader.

HAVE YOU HEARD

The following are actual bumper stickers:

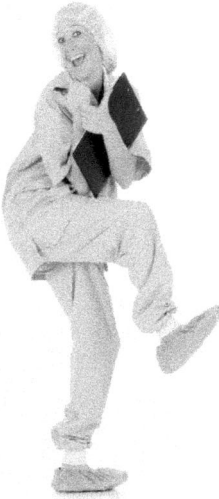

- Change is inevitable, except from a vending machine.

- Out of my mind. Back in five minutes.

- Cover me. I'm changing lanes.

- Forget about world peace. Visualize using your turn signal.

- I took an IQ test and the results were negative.

Source: www.funnymail.com

WHAT DO YOU KNOW ABOUT PREVENTING FALLS?

It helps to figure out how much you know before you start. In this way you will have an idea as to the gaps in your knowledge prior to reading the content. Please circle to indicate the best answer. Remember, at this stage, you are not expected to know all the answers:

1. Older people need the same amount of light as younger people.

a. True

b. False

2. Loose floor mats can be a risk factor for falls.

a. True

b. False

3. Reducing regular activity decreases a person's risk of falling.

a. True

b. False

4. The towel bar in the bathroom can be used as a grab bar.

a. True

b. False

5. A chair with armrests is safer than one without armrests.

a. True

b. False

6. An elderly person in your family is confused and likes to wander through the home at all times of the night. What would be an appropriate safety measure?

a. Keep him or her in bed in the highest position so she can't get out.

b. Tuck in the sheets tightly to keep him in bed.

c. Ensure the halls are safe for her to walk in.

d. Lock his bedroom door.

7. Which of the following tips would prevent falls?

a. Encouraging the person to exercise regularly.

b. Encouraging the person to hold on to the railings on the stairs.

c. Marking the edge of the steps with non-skid tape.

d. B and C.

e. A, B and C.

ANSWERS

1. b. False: Older people need more light younger people – but check out how often you find a person in a darkened room even in the day time

2. a. True: Loose mats are frequently a cause of tripping or sliding.

3. b. False: Reducing regular activity can lessen a person's general level of fitness and balance, which is so important in preventing falls.

4. b. False: A towel bar is not constructed to be strong enough to hold even average body weight.

5. a. True: Armrests on a chair can prevent a person falling sideways.

6. c. As all the other options entail restraint, your first option should be to ensure the halls are safe for her to walk.

7. d. The options b and c are commonsense tips to preventing falls.

DID YOU KNOW?

- 25% of people in the community aged 65-74 fall each year.
- 33% of people in the community aged 75 and older fall each year.
- In hospitals, 20% of older adults fall during their stay.
- In long term care facilities, 50% of residents fall each year.
- 20% of hospital admissions of older adults and 40% of admissions to long term care facilities are related to falls. This can be as high as 56% for people 75 and older.

Older adults are prone to falls, leading family members to worry about the safety of their loved ones. Falls can occur at home, in public places, or in healthcare facilities; these falls can result in serious injury or death, especially in the elderly. About 15% of falls at home result in serious injuries such as fractures. They are the leading cause of accidental death in people 79 years of age and older. Hospital stays are often longer for people who fall.

Physical injuries are not the only effects from falls. There can also be emotional effects. Falling can lead to a fear of falling again and cause a person to feel a loss of dignity. Fear of falling may reduce a person's activity, rendering them unable to care for themselves and their homes. It also causes feelings of dependency and decreases their opportunities for a fulfilling social life. Moreover, reduced activity is itself a risk factor for falling.

The major causes of falls include slippery surfaces, bad lighting, clutter, poorly fitting clothing, or improper footwear. Entrances to the home, stairs, and bathrooms can be very dangerous. Many falls are preventable. As a caregiver, you have a key role in protecting your loved one or client from falls.

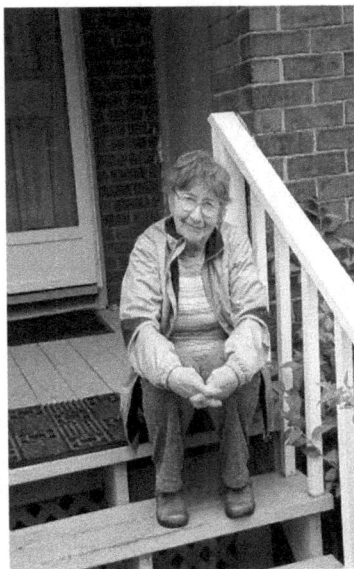

RISK FACTORS FOR FALLS

A variety of risk factors can lead to falls. You should know or have assessed your family member's or client's risk for falling. If there is a strong risk, extra things should be put into place to enhance safety.

Some risk factors can be just a normal part of aging, while others are caused by medical conditions, medications, or alcohol. Still others are caused by problems in the person's surroundings. Whatever the risk factor, there are things you can do to reduce the risk.

CONSIDER FOR A MOMENT...

Has the person you are caring for

fallen at any time?

What caused the fall?

What happened to that person

because of the fall?

AGE-RELATED FACTORS

Many changes occur as a normal part of getting older. Some of these changes increase the risk of falling.

Vision

Eyesight worsens with age. The decrease in vision increases the risk for falls. Certain eye conditions, such as cataracts or night blindness, also affect vision, making falls more likely. Older people often have difficulty telling colors apart. Seeing the edges of stairs can be a problem. Also, not being able to see small changes in the level of the floors (for example, from an area with a carpet to one without carpet) can cause people to trip and fall. Older people might not be able to see objects in their paths that could trip them.

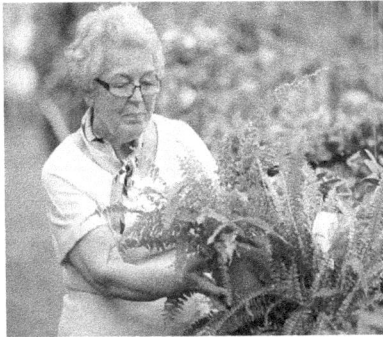

Muscle function

Muscle strength, flexibility, and range of motion in the joints decrease with age. Standing up and walking becomes more difficult to do. Weak arm muscles make it harder for some elderly people to push themselves up. It becomes harder to hold onto railings. Weak leg muscles make it harder to get up from a chair.

Balance

The elderly lose their balance more easily. Joints become stiff and bones get brittle. Older people tend not to lift their feet as much when they walk. They don't swing their arms in the same way. Reflexes slow down. Posture becomes stooped and they often lean forward when they walk.

Bathroom visits

Another normal change for many elderly people is that they need to go to the bathroom often, especially at night. They also feel a sense of urgency to get to the bathroom more quickly. Trying to get to the bathroom in the dark can increase the risk of falling. As well, if they rush to get to the bathroom, they are more likely to stumble.

OTHER FACTORS

Medical conditions

Certain medical conditions can make it more likely that older people will fall. Conditions such as arthritis cause joint stiffness. Arthritis can lead to problems holding objects and moving around. Other medical conditions can cause people to lean forward to keep their balance or to shuffle while walking. Still other illnesses can lead to brittle bones and decreased feeling in the feet and lower legs.

Medications

Medications can be a major cause of falls. Certain medications cause decreased vision, confusion, memory loss, weakness, drowsiness, and dizziness. Adjusting or changing the medication may solve the problem.

Alcohol use

Consuming alcohol can also lead to falls. The risk increases when an older person, who is taking medication, drinks alcohol. Your family member or client should be notified of the possible impact on their safety and health when they take medications and also consume alcohol.

Walking aids

Canes and walkers that are not used properly can also increase the risk for falls. As well, these aids must fit properly.

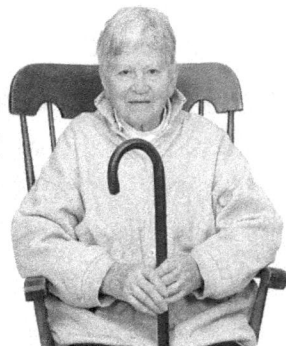

Psychosocial issues

Psychosocial problems can be risk factors. When people are depressed and lonely, they tend to get out and about much less than usual. A fear of falling, especially after a previous fall, can also lead to decreased activity. As mentioned earlier, decreased activity puts the older person at greater risk of falling.

Caregiver issues

Several risk factors stem from the caregiver. These include delays in responding to requests, delays in answering call bells, improper use of restraints, unsafe transfer practices, and poor supervision of the people in their care.

ENVIRONMENTAL FACTORS

The environment can have safety features that protect against falls. Common safety features include good lighting, handrails on stairs, grab bars in the bathroom, and non-slip mats in the bathtub.

The environment can also be filled with dangers that can lead to falls. Hazards may include:

- wet floors
- loose floor rugs that can slide on the floor
- furniture that tips easily
- furniture that is difficult to get out of
- telephone or electrical cords that hang and can trip an older person
- clutter or objects in areas where the person walks
- using high shelves or cupboards requiring step stools
- stairs that are broken or do not have railings
- cracks or broken sections in outside walkways
- broken gutters that leak water onto outside walkways

- high furniture (beds, chairs)
- unsafe clothing – poor fitting shoes and socks, inappropriate footwear (wearing slippers outside), long robes or pant legs, and dangling cords or hems

Many other risk factors may be present in the environment. Young pets that jump and move quickly underfoot can be a problem. Older people who move to unfamiliar surroundings may be at increased risk. Other examples of risks are restraints (fighting against their use) and side rails (climbing over them).

CONSIDER FOR A MOMENT...

Think about other elderly relatives
who have fallen.

What risk factors applied to them?

Does he/she have any risk factors?

TIPS TO AVOID FALLS

Stay healthy

One of the best tips for avoiding falls is for older people to stay as healthy as possible. Encourage family members or clients to take steps to promote their own health. Older people should make sure they are eating well. Good nutrition and adequate fluids are important.

Good vision

Make sure your family member has his or her eyes checked regularly. Glasses should be kept clean and worn as needed. Regular visits to physicians and health professionals are important. With regular visits, medical conditions can be managed. Side effects of medications can also be controlled.

Appropriate exercise

Encourage your loved one or client to be as active and independent as possible. However, rushing should be avoided when doing activities. Older people should maintain balance, strength, joints, muscles, posture, and walking pattern by exercising regularly.

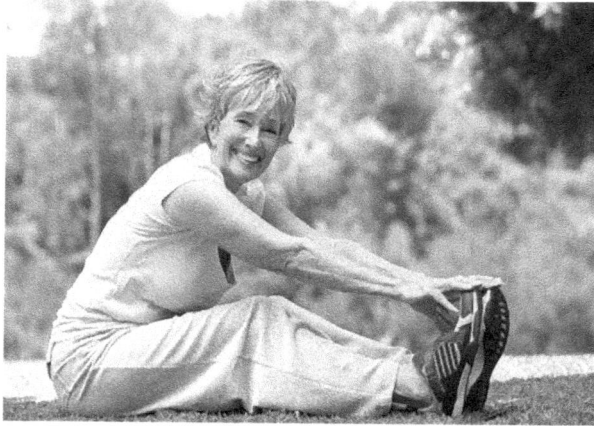

Regular exercise makes the older person feel stronger and healthier. Even little things can help. A client or loved one can squeeze a ball to improve grip. Lifting their arms over their head while sitting will help joints and muscles. If necessary, provide assistance and support for older people when they walk. Use walkers or canes to assist with walking. However, make sure your client or family member is properly fitted for the walker or cane. Make sure they know how to use it correctly. Canes and walkers should have non-slip bottoms. Consult healthcare professionals for special exercises and special equipment as needed.

Safety tips

Teach the older person simple moves to increase safety. When bending, place feet apart and bend from the knees. Do not turn quickly. Carry small loads. Small loads won't block vision and won't put the person off balance.

Appropriate clothing

Ensure clothes are of proper length. Long robes or pants can be tripped over. There should not be any dangling cords or hems. Footwear should be safe and appropriate, it should fit properly, and have good support. Footwear should have non-skid soles and flat, broad heels. Appropriate means wearing the right kind of shoe for the surroundings. For example, slippers should not be worn outside.

HOME CHECKLIST

What is in the home that can increase the risk of falling? Here are some things you should look for:

Lighting

How good is the lighting? An 85-year-old needs about three times as much light as a 15-year-old to see the same thing. This is especially important on stairs, entrances, and walkways. Lampshades or frosted bulbs reduce glare. Is there a light next to the bed? The older person should be able to turn the light on and off without getting out of bed. Are there any nightlights? Are flashlights distributed throughout the house, especially on different levels? These will be needed if the electricity goes out.

Furniture

What is the furniture like? Where is it positioned? Arrange furniture so it's easy to get around. Move low tables away from where the older person will be walking. This prevents the person from falling over the table. Older people often lean on furniture as they try to stand or walk. Furniture that could topple should be positioned away from where the older person is walking. Sturdy furniture is easier to get out of. Boards placed under cushions and mattresses will make them firmer. Furniture with armrests is also easier to get out of. Cover or cushion sharp corners on furniture or cupboards. Talk to your family member or client about having all unnecessary furniture removed.

Floors and stairs

The use of stairs in general can lead to increased risk of falls. Slippery stairs in particular can be very dangerous. Assist loved ones or clients to arrange their living space to avoid stairs as much as possible.

Are there hand rails on the stairs? Are the hand rails in good condition? This is important for stairs and steps inside and outside the house. Contrasting colors are easier to see so different colors should be used as much as possible.

Step care

Use different-colored paint or non-skid tape on the edges of steps. This will help the person to see the edge of the stairs. Consider painting the first and last step a different color. If needed, use safety gates at the top of stairs. However, ensure your loved one or client does not try to climb over the gate.

Clutter-free areas

Remove things that can be tripped over from walking areas and stairs. Examples are clothes, books, and shoes. Many people place items that have to be brought upstairs on the bottom of the stairs.

Prevent slipping

Are the floors slippery? Use non-skid flooring and non-skid floor wax. Clean up spills quickly. Tape loose mats and rugs down with double-sided tape or remove them. Use a non-slip mat in front of the kitchen sink. Are leaks present? Leaks can make walking areas slippery. Is there a glare on the floor? A glare can make it difficult for people to see the floor. A non-glare wax can be used if necessary to correct the problem.

Level surfaces

Did you ever notice that older people tend not to lift their feet very high as they walk? Because of this, floor surfaces at different levels can cause them to trip. For example, one part of the floor can be carpeted and another part uncarpeted resulting in uneven surfaces. Are there any torn sections in the carpets? Are there any cracks or broken areas in walkways? The thresholds in doorways may be lower than the area around them. All of these things can cause tripping.

Bathrooms

Many falls take place in the bathroom. Older people often rush to get to the bathroom or they may try to get to the bathroom in the dark during the night. They may have trouble getting on and off the toilet. They may have difficulty getting in and out of the bathtub or shower. The bathtub or shower can have a slippery surface. Are there proper grab bars or handrails in the bathroom? Hand rails should be near the toilet and bathtub. Encourage your family member or client not to use the towel bar. Towel bars are often not strong enough to support the person.

Bathroom organization

Are there non-slip mats or strips in the bathtub or shower? Is there a seat or bench in the shower or bathtub? Are the soap, shampoo, and towel within easy reach without stretching or bending? Can your loved one or client get in and out of the bathtub or shower easily?

Toilet seat

Does the older person have difficulty getting on and off the toilet? A raised toilet seat might help.

Frequent visits

Encourage your family member to use the bathroom regularly. This will help to avoid rushing to get to the bathroom. Are nightlights used?

Dangerous cords

Are electrical cords or telephone cords dangling? These can be tripped over.

Glass doors

Are there any glass doors in the house? Placing colored tape on the door will make the door easier to see.

Reaching objects

Are objects that are used often easily reached? Overreaching, climbing on stools, chairs, and ladders, and bending over for objects might lead to falls. Encourage the use of object-reaching devices. If ladders must be used, ensure they are sturdy.

Telephone issues

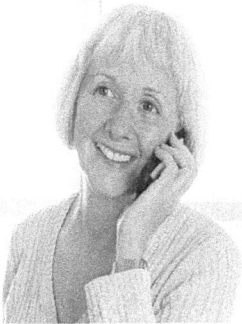

Are there telephones throughout the house, especially on different levels? Talk to your family member or client about using cordless telephones. Is the phone within easy reach from the floor? If a fall occurs, the client may not be able to stand up. Have emergency phone numbers programmed into the phone. If your loved one or client is prone to falling, some type of personal alarm in case of a fall may be needed.

Outside the home

The same strategies should be used outside the house. Is the lighting good? Do the steps have railings? Are the edges of the steps easily seen? Are the steps and walkways in good condition? Are there any garden tools or clutter in walkways? Suggest that your client of family member wear a hat and sunglasses to help reduce the glare from the sun.

CONSIDER FOR A MOMENT...

Remember the activity you did

a few minutes ago.

You listed possible risk factors

around your home.

Now that you've completed

this section, think about it again.

Can you add any more risk

factors to your list?

FALLS PREVENTION IN
HEALTHCARE FACILITIES

Your family member may be residing in a health care facility and it is a fact that falls among older clients in healthcare facilities are a serious problem. Studies have shown that about half of the older clients in healthcare institutions fall each year.

Apply all of the tips that we have discussed so far to prevent falls in healthcare facilities as well. Safe footwear, safe bathrooms, safe stairs, and good lighting are still important. However, healthcare facilities have some special concerns. Surroundings are unfamiliar. Routines are different. Different equipment is used. Older people often have more medical conditions that can make them prone to falls.

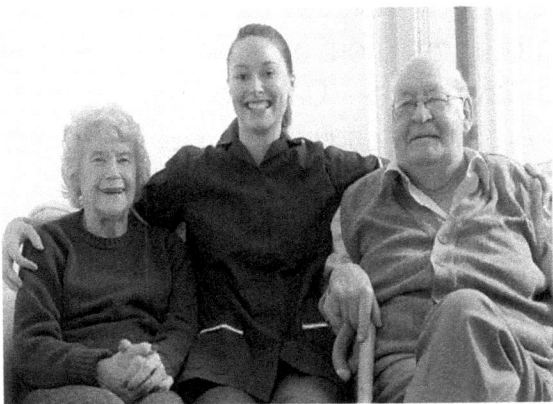

You should try to make sure that you champion your family member's integration into a health care facility to address and minimize the risks. Here are some of the issues that the health care facility should address for your family member:

Provide an introduction

Ensure your loved one is shown around the unit when they are first admitted. If the older person is at risk for falls make sure her room is as close to the nursing station as possible.

Identify high risk clients

Facilities usually have a policy to carefully monitor clients for their risk of falling. They look for signs of dizziness, weakness, drowsiness, fatigue, or loss of balance. They should pay attention while clients are walking or carrying out other activities. Can they go up and down stairs? Can they get up from chairs easily? Are they steady when they bend over? The staff must be vigilant regarding these issues.

Encourage independence

Facilities should encourage clients to be as active and independent as possible. They should teach your family member how to transfer safely from bed to chair or from chair to toilet. They should also consult with health professionals for specific exercises and equipment as needed.

Safety tips

Are the bedside table and frequently used items placed near the client? Are the wheels locked on beds and chairs? Is the bed kept in its lowest position? Keeping the bed low whenever you leave a client who is at risk for falls may help to prevent injuries. Is broken equipment repaired promptly? Is the client's room free of clutter? Many facilities have railings running along the hallways; clients should be encouraged to hold onto these railings as they walk.

Call bell

Is there a call bell within easy reach? Clients should be encouraged to use them. Even though healthcare facilities wants their clients to be as independent as possible, they should encourage your family member to ask for assistance when needed. Call bells should always be answered as quickly as possible.

Special considerations

Your loved one may be confused and may wander. He or she requires a safe environment and close supervision. Healthcare workers should monitor all activities and remove unsafe objects. There are also safety devices that can be used to prevent falls. Pressure alarms can be used on chairs and beds. There are leg bands with monitoring sensors available – when a client tries to get out of bed or a chair, the change in pressure will trigger an alarm.

SIDE RAILS

Side rails can prevent falls for some older people. Sometimes, however, using side rails may not be the safest option for your family member.

You will not have to decide whether side rails should or should not be used. This is a decision that should be made by healthcare professionals. If side rails are being used with your family member, ask the facility why that is – what is it about your loved one's condition that requires the use of side rails?

Side rails may be used with family members who are sedated or unconscious. They may be used with an older person who is at risk of rolling out of bed. Side rails may be used with confused family members. They may be used with your family member who needs assistance to get up and walk. The health care facility often hopes the side rails will remind the older person not to try to get up without assistance. However, this does not always work.

Elderly people who are smaller than average can get trapped between the side rails and the bed, or a part of their body can get caught. A confused person may attempt to climb out over the side rails. Moreover, many older people may view the side rails as barriers, which can make them feel afraid or confined.

The facility will use side rails if the client's condition calls for them – for instance, if a client is unconscious. Leaving one side rail up may serve to remind your family member about the best side to use when he or she gets out of bed. Padded rails may help if an older person gets himself or part of his body trapped between the rails. Bed alarms may help to notify staff if a person tries to climb out over the rails.

Trying to predict a client's needs may help to prevent her from climbing over the rails. It might also be a way to avoid using rails in some cases. The healthcare facility staff should always assist clients to get out of bed and to a chair before the person tries to do it herself and risks falling. Staff should also assist clients to the lounge or dining room.

The need to go to the bathroom is a frequent reason for getting out of bed. The staff should assist clients to the bathroom regularly and should answer call bells promptly.

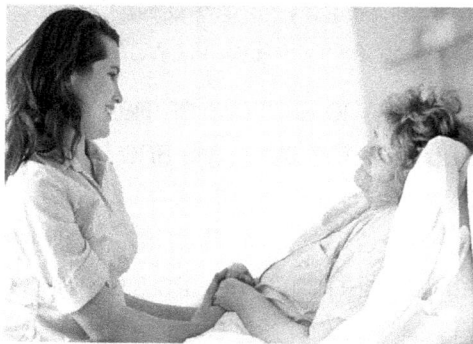

RESTRAINTS

A restraint is something that restricts movement. It can be a physical restraint, such as a vest, belt or wrist restraint. These are used to tie the older person to a certain place. Side rails can also be a type of physical restraint. There are chemical restraints, too, such as drugs which can be used to sedate a client.

Restraints should be used only when absolutely necessary. It has been shown that restraints do not guarantee client safety and can lead to injuries. They can cause physical harm, loss of dignity, and even death. Some of the problems include:

- breathing problems from vests that have not been properly applied
- problems with blood flow
- damage to skin
- loss of muscle tone and broken bones
- difficulty eating and drinking
- problems with toileting

> **CONSIDER FOR A MOMENT...**
>
> What safety features or
> safety policies are in place
> in the facility where your
> family member is living?

Sometimes facilities use restraints in particular situations. These are the guidelines when restraints are used.

- The staff should know the facility's policy regarding restraints.

- A physician or healthcare professional will need to make this decision about using restraints. The decision should be based on the older person's current condition, not what happened in the past. The possibility of injury, both to the family member and to others, should also be considered.

- Caregivers need to be aware of restraints being used with their loved one.
- The staff should try other measures first such as:
  - Involve family members in the client's care as much as possible.
  - Try to determine why the problem is occurring. Does the family member need to go to the bathroom? Is he/she confused? Afraid? Can anything be done to fix the problem?
  - Provide a soothing environment. Reduce noise. Play music that the client enjoys. Use a nightlight. Make the surroundings as homelike as possible.
  - Allow restless older people to walk around in a safe area.
  - Encourage exercise and activity. Allow the older person to assist with tasks.
  - Make sure the older person is assisted to the bathroom often.
  - Use non-restraint safety devices if available. These include pressure alarms in the beds or chairs or in leg bands worn by the client. When the pressure changes, such as when the client tries to get out of bed, an alarm goes off.

- The least restrictive type of restraint should be used to meet the older person's needs. To keep the older person's dignity, it should be concealed from others as much as possible.

- The staff should check the older person and the restraint frequently according to the facility's policy.

- Remove the restraints regularly according to the facility's policy.

- Chart the necessary information according to the facility's policy.

WHAT TO DO IF AN OLDER PERSON FALLS

When a fall occurs, stay with the family member until help comes. If you suspect an injury, don't try to move him or her on your own. Have your loved one assessed by a healthcare professional. If your family member falls in a facility, the staff should follow facility policies. They will know who to notify and the forms to complete and will write down the details of the fall.

Most healthcare facilities have a policy that requires staff to complete an incident report form when a fall occurs. (Some facilities have different names for these forms but they all serve a similar purpose.) These forms document important information about the fall such as the date and time and details of the event. Quite often patterns related to the falls can be found once the information is examined. For example, one facility discovered that a certain elderly female client fell only in the early morning when attempting to get to the bathroom on her own. The problem resolved once staff started routinely taking her to the bathroom each morning before she had a chance to try and go on her own.

CONSIDER FOR A MOMENT...

What does the facility's policy
say it should do if an
older person falls?
If you're not sure, find out.

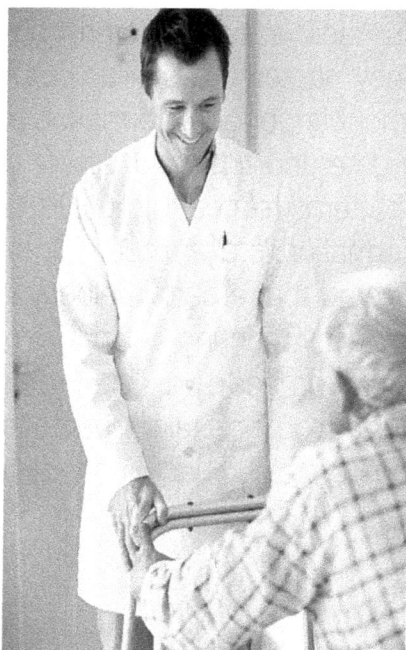

CASE EXAMPLE

Mrs. Bagley is 71 years old. She lives alone. She may be similar to your loved one.

Each time you visit her, you notice that Mrs. Bagley appears a little more frail. She now frequently stumbles a little as she walks. You also notice a large bruise on her lower left leg. She tells you that the bruise appeared after she fell in the bathroom a couple of days ago. What should you do?

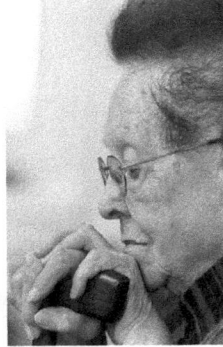

YOUR ANSWERS TO CASE EXAMPLE

SUGGESTED ANSWERS TO CASE EXAMPLE

Immediate priorities

You will need to find out whether a healthcare professional has seen her recently. Has she been assessed for an injury since the fall?

Find out what her risk factors for falls are.

• How often has she fallen?

• Does she have regular activity?

• Does she use a cane or walker?

• Does she wear glasses?

• Does she wear appropriate footwear?

• Are her clothes too long?

• Does she have dangling hems or cords?

Look around her home.

• Is the lighting good?

• What safety features are present in her home?

• What are the hazards that could lead to falls?

• Pay special attention to the bathroom, stairs, and floors.

• What about outside areas? Are they safe?

Depending upon what you find, you may be able to suggest tips that will help to avoid future falls:

- Make sure she wears safe footwear.

- Encourage her to wear her glasses.

- Make sure the lighting is good throughout the house.

- Ensure there is nothing on the floors or stairs that could cause her to trip.

- Suggest grab bars in the bathroom and a non-slip mat in the bathtub.

This is only a sample of some of the tips you might consider for your possible situation.

CONCLUSION

Falls occur often, especially with older people. Falls can occur at home, in public places, or health care facilities. These falls can cause serious injuries or death. However, falls can be prevented. By learning about the risk factors for falls and the strategies to prevent them, you can help to prevent falls among your family members.

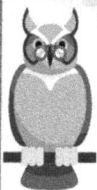

CHECK YOUR KNOWLEDGE

1. Identify 4 age-related risk factors for falls.

2. What risk factors would you look for in an older person's home?

3. What can you do to improve safety on stairs?

4. Identify 4 tips to improve safety in bathrooms.

5. What are the problems with using side rails?

6. Describe other strategies that can be used instead of restraints.

7. What should you do if someone in your care does fall?

TEST YOURSELF

Please circle to indicate the best answer:

1. Only older people with medical conditions are at risk of falling.

a. True

b. False

2. Restraints should not always be used with people at risk for falls.

a. True

b. False

3. Older people at risk for falls should be in rooms near the nursing station.

a. True

b. False

4. Trying to get to the bathroom is a frequent cause of falls.

a. True

b. False

5. Side rails always prevent falls.

a. True

b. False

6. Which of the following increases the safety in the bathroom?

a. Encourage the person to hold onto the towel rack.

b. Ensure the soap and towel are within easy reach.

c. Use a non-slip mat in the bathtub.

d. B and C

e. A, B, and C

7. You are in an older person's home. Which of the following would you consider to be a risk factor for falls?

a. The person wears knitted slippers or socks on the vinyl flooring in the kitchen.

b. The person uses an object-reaching device for high cupboards.

c. The person has the top and bottom step painted a different color.

d. The person uses frosted light bulbs.

ANSWERS

1. b. False. Some risk factors are related to the older person while some can be just a normal part of aging. Others are caused by medical conditions, medications, or alcohol. Still others are caused by problems in the client's surroundings.

2. a. True. Restraints should be used only if absolutely necessary.

3. a. True. Older people at risk for falls should be placed in rooms as close to the nursing station as possible.

4. a. True. Trying to get to the bathroom in the dark can increase the risk of falling. As well, if they rush to get to the bathroom, they are more likely to stumble.

5. b. False. Small people can get trapped between the side rails and the bed, or a body part can get caught. A confused person may climb out over the side rails. And many older people may view the side rails as barriers, which can make them feel afraid or confined.

6. d. Always ensure the soap and towel are within easy reach and use a non-slip mat in the bathtub.

7. a. Knitted slippers or socks can slip on vinyl flooring.

REFERENCES

Capezuti, E., Talerico, K.A., Cochran, I., Becker, H. Strumpf, N. & Evans, L. (1999). Individualized interventions to prevent bed-related falls and reduce siderail use. Journal of Gerontological Nursing, 25(11), 26-34.

Craven, R.F., & Hirnle, C. J. (2000). Fundamentals of nursing: Human health and function (3rd ed., pp. 644-649). Philadelphia, PA: Lippincott.

Department of Human Services, Government of Victoria. (2000). Preventing falls among older people. Retrieved January 17, 2002 from http://www.dhs.vic. gov.au/acmh/aged/maintaining/falls.htm

Eliopoulos, C. (2001). Gerontological nursing (5th ed., pp. 143-145). Philadelphia, PA: Lippincott.

Kozier, B., Erb, G., Berman, A., & Burke, K. (2000). Fundamentals of nursing: Concepts, process, and practice (6th ed., pp. 679-681). Upper Saddle River, NJ: Prentice Hall Health.

Meyer, M., & Derr, P. (1998). Preparing the home. The comfort of home: An illustrated step-by-step guide for caregivers (pp. 92-113). Portland, Oregon: CareTrust Publications.

Miller, C.A. (1999). Mobility and safety. Nursing care of older adults – Theory & practice (3rd ed., pp. 343-374). Philadelphia, PA: Lippincott.

National Center for Injury Prevention and Control. (1998). Preventing falls among seniors. Retrieved from January 17, 2002 from http://www.cdc.gov. ncipc/duip/spotlite/falls.htm

Rawsky, E. (1998). Review of literature on falls among the elderly. Image – The Journal of Nursing Scholarship, 30(1), 47-52.

Safer Community Advocate – Maribyrnong City Council. (1999-2000). Maribyrnong falls prevention program. Retrieved February 6, 2002 http:// infowest.maribyrnong.vic.gov.au/fallsprevention/html/abou.htm

Stolley, J.M., Lewis, A., Moore, L. & Harvey, P. (2001). Risk for Injury: Falls. In M.L. Maas, K.C. Buckwalter, M.D. Hardy, T. Tripp-Reimer, M.G. Titler, & J.P. Specht. (2001). Nursing care of older adults: Diagnoses, outcomes, & interventions (pp. 23-33). St. Louis, Missouri: Mosby.

Sullivan, G. (1999). Minimizing your risk in patient falls. RN, 62(4), 69-72.

Taylor, C., Lillis, C., & LeMone, P. (2001). Fundamentals of nursing: The art & science of nursing care (4th ed., pp. 516-520). Philadelphia, PA: Lippincott.

Walker, A. (2001). Preventing falls at home. Nursing Communities: Home Health. Retrieved December 19, 2001 from http://www.springnet.com/homehealth/hh074.htm

Walker, B. (1998). Preventing falls. RN, 61(5), 40-42.

Winslow, E., & Jacobson, A. (1998). Reducing falls in older patients. American Journal of Nursing, 98(10), 22.